The Journey of Weight loss and Fitness

Why you shouldn't keep that excess fat and remain fit

BLOOM DELMA

DEDICATION

I dedicate this book to my family. They've been my support through each
book I write

CONTENTS

INTRODUCTION

 Hello, my name is Blossom and for years I thought that losing weight was also the same as keeping fit. Lord knows I tried so many diets, so many exercises, so many waist trainers. But guess what? I did not lose weight nor did I become fit.

I kept on trying different things till I finally found the one thing that worked for me. I didn't need a specialist to tell me that maintenance would be the problem, but there's this thing about habits that they say, "Once you try something for 21 days consistently, it becomes a part of you".

My fitness and weight loss journey.

I'm sure by now you're wondering what I did or what I'm doing, that's the point of this book.

But before we continue I want to tell you a little story.

Right from high school or secondary school, I've always been slim, I weighed nothing more than 55kg or 121pounds. In your mind you're wondering why I wrote this book or where the weight came from, we're getting there.

I was an athlete, I played soccer, basketball, and volleyball. If you noticed, I used past tense, why? The moment I left high school I stopped every form of sport because there was no time for it again.

I started gaining weight, at first, it would be 2kg or 4.4pounds, I'd wave it off and continue my life. Till I started stress eating, eating more snacks than food, taking a lot of beverages and I forgot that in my family we tend to be fat and what's worse is it's hard to lose the weight gain in my family.

Before I knew it, I weighed 87kg or 191.8kg.

Obesity, the horror.

Insecurity became my name. Someone who was once comfortable in her skin hated her body and that's when I tried all sorts of things but nothing worked.

My metabolism is slow which means that my body needs fewer calories to keep on going which also means my body burns fewer calories, which means more gets stored as fat in the body.

I saw the signs, for example, I was exhausted every time, I constantly had headaches even when I wasn't stressed, I added weight and so many more signs but I refused to take heed because I saw it as not necessary.

At this point, I still didn't know that I had a slow metabolism.

One thing you need to know is that metabolism plays a minor role. From research, poor diet and inactivity are the major causes.

After a while, I just gave up on the dream of losing weight till something miraculous happened and now it's just the maintenance that we're working on because even if you lose weight, one little thing can make you withdraw and gain everything you suffered to lose.

On that note, let's get right into the book.

FITNESS

Fitness can mean different things to different people.

According to the dictionary, fitness is the condition of being fit, suitable, or appropriate.

I'm sure this is more confusing than what you already have in mind.

"For me, fitness is first and foremost about feeling good and being able to move without pain," says the certified strength and conditioning specialist Grayson Wickham, a New York City-based physical therapist and the founder of Movement Vault, a mobility, and movement company. He explains that true fitness is about feeling healthy and being in sufficient shape to do the activities you want to do and live the lifestyle you want to live.

To be fit, you have to do things that you normally do that would make you all winded up or out of breath or in need of a break.

For example, walking up the stairs, I noticed that when I was fat, I always needed to breathe halfway through. Walking up a hill, hiking and so many other examples you can think of.

Fitness is a state of balance physically and emotionally.

It's an attitude toward your health and wellness.

Traditionally, experts have defined five key components of physical fitness:

•Body composition (the relative proportion of fat and fat-free tissue in the body),

•Cardiorespiratory or aerobic fitness,

•Flexibility,

•Muscular strength and

•Muscular endurance.

But let's not forget the impact of nutrition, sleep, and mental and emotional health on fitness either.

Reduction in these things can cause a detriment to your total well-being.

So how do you make fitness part of your overall lifestyle — and reach your individual fitness goals?

Research shows that aerobic exercise is important for cardiovascular health (the intensity you choose should be based on your current fitness level and your doctor's recommendations).

 Examples include walking, running, cycling, and swimming.

Strength workouts should target one or all of the body's basic muscle groups, such as the legs, core, back, hips, chest, or arms.

Lifting weights, working with resistance bands, or performing body-weight exercises are all good options and should be used to match, and improve, your current fitness level.

That may sound overwhelming but not if you expand how you think of exercise beyond time spent in the gym.

Wickham says instead, think about all the movement you do as exercise.

Some movement is better than none, and no matter how short a spurt of activity is, it can still count toward your weekly goals. The bottom line is that adults should be moving more and sitting less for the rest of their days.

Facts about fitness that you never knew:

•The human body has 650 muscles.

•The heart is the strongest muscle in the body.

•Nearly 50% of all young people ages 12-21 are not vigorously active daily.

•For every pound of muscle gained, the body burns 50 extra calories every day.

•Only 13% of men are physically fit.

•Exercise makes you feel more energized because it releases endorphins into the blood.

•Movement in exercise helps relieve stress by producing a relaxation response which serves as a position distraction.

WEIGHT LOSS

The dictionary definition of weight loss is the reduction of total body mass due to the loss of fluids, fat, tissues, and so on.

The point is from the definition we can see clearly that fitness and weight loss aren't the same, I mean we're still going to discuss that but that's just the beginning.

You don't need me to tell you that losing weight — and keeping it off — is hard. But understanding why weight loss is so difficult can help you stop beating yourself up over every little setback, and increase your chances of success.

•Your body works against you: When you try to lose weight, you're fighting not only your cravings but also your own body. Weight loss decreases the hormone leptin, which signals to your brain that you're full, and increases the hormone ghrelin, which stimulates hunger, Australian researchers found. This hormone imbalance continues long after you succeed at weight loss, making it even harder for you to keep the pounds off, according to the study.

Plus, if you cut too many calories too quickly, your

metabolism will slow. Eating too little also makes you more likely to rebound and go in the opposite direction by overeating because you were restricting yourself for so long. I recommend doing things more moderately: Increasing physical activity and decreasing calories are what work in the long run.

•There Are No Quick Fixes:

When you're trying to lose weight, it's hard to be patient. But avoid the temptation to try something drastic. Since quick starvation diets can wreak havoc on your metabolism, they can damage your weight loss efforts in the long term. As you start your diet, remember that slow and steady weight loss — or one to two pounds a week — is the easiest to maintain.

To lose a pound of fat, you have to burn 3,500 calories more than you consume, so you can see how hard it is to exercise your way through a poor diet. Instead, you have to watch what you eat and exercise. If there's any "magic" to dieting, it's in that combination.

•Diet Supplements:

Those little pills that claim to supercharge your metabolism are tempting, but there's little evidence that they work. In a review published in May 2012 in the American Journal of Preventive Medicine, researchers at Beth Israel Deaconess Medical Center in Boston followed thousands of dieters and found that liquid diets, fad diets, and over-the-counter diet pills were not linked to weight loss. So what worked? Eating less fat, exercising more, using prescription weight loss medication, and joining commercial weight loss programs.

•One Diet Doesn't Fit All:

Everyone's body is unique, so the diet that works for your friend, your coworker, your mother, or your sister might not work for you. When looking at how best to lose weight, consider your health and family history, your metabolism, your activity level, your age, your gender, and your likes and dislikes. When you're dieting, it's important to allow yourself some foods that you enjoy or else you'll feel deprived and be less likely to stick with an overall healthy eating plan. For weight loss success, tailor your diet to your body and accept that one diet won't work for everyone.

•Cardio Is Essential (and Strength Training Helps too):

According to the 2018 Physical Activity Guidelines for Americans, published in November 2018 in the Journal of the American Medical Association, adults should get 150 minutes of moderate-intensity aerobic exercise, or 75 minutes of vigorous aerobic activity (or a combination of both), preferably spread throughout the week, plus two or more days of muscle-strengthening activities. And every bit counts — the recommendation is to move more throughout the day, even if it's just a walk around the block.

These guidelines should help most people lose weight, but obese people or people with a lot of weight to lose the need to be even more active, working up to at least 30 minutes per day over time. Plus, don't skip the strength training. Increased muscle mass also gives your metabolism a slight boost — and makes you look more sleek and svelte.

•He Can Eat More Than She Can:

It doesn't seem fair, but men can eat more than women and still lose weight. That's because men tend to naturally burn more calories than women, thanks to their larger size, muscle mass, and elevated levels of the hormone testosterone, which promotes muscle growth. Plus, the male body is genetically designed for more muscle and less fat than the female body because men do not have to store the energy required to bear children. Once you come to terms with this fact and start eating less than your male partner or friends, the scale will thank you.

•It's Not a Diet, It's a Lifestyle Change:

If you want to lose weight and keep it off, you have to change your behavior not just until you reach your goal weight, but for the months and years to follow. That's because as soon as you stop your "diet," you're likely to gain back the pounds you worked so hard to shed. To be successful at weight loss, you need to make sustainable lifestyle changes, like making healthy food choices at almost every meal, and getting plenty of exercises every week (https://www.everydayhealth.com/weight-pictures/hard-truths-about-weight-loss.aspx).

Create your plan to lose weight based on BMI, height, age, daily activity, and habits. And if you can't you can click on the link below, trust me this is one of the best ways to lose weight.

https://unimeal.com/final-ntrl/e02f9fed-1130-485d-b2b3-ff24094df60b?pricing=1

THE DIFFERENCE BETWEEN FITNESS AND WEIGHT LOSS

From the title, I'm sure we have an idea of where I'm going with this.

Without further ado, when you start a weight loss journey, your goal is basically to go on a diet and shed weight.

But when you exercise, your aim is wide, you can either do it to lose weight, to gain weight, or even for your overall health.

Diet just means eating healthy, lower-calorie meals. Exercise means being more physically active. Although people appropriately focus on diet when they're trying to lose weight, being active also is an essential component of weight loss but we tend to ignore that and continue our weight loss journey like that.

Note that if you diet without working out, you'll end up losing weight, it's true. But if you've lost weight without exercise, it may be because you're losing muscle mass. Second, your stress hormones may have leveled out plus the diet you're probably on and as a result, led to weight loss.

Now don't get me wrong, it's beautiful to lose weight without exercise, honestly.

But if your goal is weight loss, you should prioritize diet over exercise because it will have a much larger impact. If your time is limited, consider resistance training (rather than cardio) to help maintain your muscle mass and metabolic rate or HIIT to help you achieve a similar calorie burn as cardio in less time.

But for people who are obese, first of all, you're beautiful just the way you are. Secondly, losing weight might be more important to your overall health than focusing on fitness. In fact, evidence shows that exercise alone is not an effective way to lose weight. Rather, effective weight loss is mostly about what you eat, though it should also include exercise.

Exercise helps prolong your life and maintain the weight you have after you've lost it.

Finally, if you're gaining weight even while you're on a diet, you may be eating more calories than your body is using. Calories play a big role in controlling your weight.

REASONS WHY YOU NEED TO BE FIT

The end is near but what can I say? This journey is as stressful as it can get, but the result is worth it.

Because fitness is the state of being physically able to live the happy, fulfilling life you want — the first and most obvious payoff of achieving fitness is a high quality of life.

The following are some reasons why you should be fit:

•Exercise is helpful for weight loss and maintaining weight loss.

•Exercise can increase metabolism, or how many calories you burn in a day.

•It can also help you maintain and increase lean body mass, which also helps increase the number of calories you burn each day.

•Increased energy levels.

•Better work-life balance.

•Stronger immunity.

•Sounder sleep.

•Some research suggests that increasing your fitness through exercise may help mild to moderate depression just as much as medication.

•Physical activity is also connected to better focus and productivity. Because exercise increases the flow of blood and oxygen to the brain.

•When your body becomes fitter, it lengthens its chromosomes' protective caps, called telomeres.

•Thosetelomeres is in charge of determining how quickly your cells age. That means keeping them in top shape (being fit) can help lengthen your life span.

CONCLUSION

You may not notice many of the greatest benefits of fitness for years or even decades but you'll need patience.

I studied my body over the years as I grew and I realized that eating more when I'm physically active would help me lose weight fast. When I say I was physically active I mean I did a lot of walks, and a lot of climbing up and down the stairs, I didn't actively find a routine for exercise.

And I did a lot of fasting. During the space of when I'd eat, it would always be much cause I was physically active.

But then I got conscious of my weight when I stopped being physically active, all I did was portion control.

If you want to lose weight without exercising, simply reducing your portion size can be a big help. Combined with eating slowly and drinking lots of water, taking this simple step can allow you to reduce calories and drop weight but you need the willpower to do this, especially if this is your first time.

Why is weight loss so hard? You might ask.

I did some research and found out that losing weight triggers biological mechanisms that make it harder to keep the weight off — including a slower metabolism. The more effort you put into losing weight, the more you can stretch that spring out — that is, lose weight.

Your weight is a balance between the calories you take in and the calories you burn. You will lose weight if you burn off more calories than you take in, and you will gain weight if you eat more calories than you burn off.

That's all you need to know about weight loss, next time I'll talk about something that relates to our health but is highly overlooked or highly misused.